THE

COLLAGEN BOOK

With Bonus Section on PDO Threads

JAMES McHALE, D.C.

"If there is magic on this planet, it is contained in water."

—Loren Eisely

This statement may or may not be true—it is not for me to determine.

But I know that there is, most definitely, magic in the 8744 Clubhouse in Levittown, PA. I found it to be a place of transformation, love, support, action, and kindness. Many thanks to all of my friends and family who have loved, encouraged, and supported me this past year. I hope that the opportunities arise to allow me to repay this great debt.

A bucket full of thanks to Erica J., Shannon C., and Siobhan E for all of their support and encouragement during the painstaking eight months required to write this book. My apologies if I had been "less than present" when you needed me. But I am grateful that all of you stepped into the gap in an effort to help me achieve my goal of finishing my first book. I would encourage the reader to find yourself a bright, goal oriented, dedicated, loyal Erica J., Shannon C., and a Siobhan E. and maybe, just maybe, I'll be reading your book one day. And that would be very good.

Warmest Wishes for health, love, and happiness!

James McHale, D.C.
Author

Www.thecollagenbook.com
thecollagenbook@gmail.com

CONTENTS

CHAPTER 1
Introduction to Collagen

Collagen, an intricate and abundant protein in the human body, plays a pivotal role in supporting our various tissues and organs. Boasting a unique triple helix structure, collagen has multiple forms, with over 28 different types identified in the human body. These types contribute significantly to tissues such as skin, bone, and cartilage. Beyond providing structural support, collagen promotes cell growth and differentiation and facilitates wound healing. Age, genetics, lifestyle habits, and environmental factors can all impact the production of this vital protein. This chapter sets the foundation for understanding collagen, its types, structure, and importance, offering insights crucial for those seeking health and beauty benefits.

Collagen: The Body's Binding Protein

Often described as the body's "glue," the term collagen derives from the Greek word "kólla." This foundational protein ensures the cohesion, elasticity, and regeneration of all our connective tissues, effectively "holding us together." Not only is collagen essential for the integrity of our skin, bones, and joints, but it also plays a pivotal role in maintaining muscle mass and metabolism, making collagen-based supplements increasingly popular.

Peering into Peptides: Collagen Peptides Explained

Collagen peptides, commonly referred to as hydrolyzed collagen, are fragments derived from animal collagen broken down via hydrolysis. This process enhances the bioavailability of collagen, ensuring our bodies can absorb it more effectively. By contributing to new collagen production and repairing existing structures, these peptides offer a plethora of health benefits, from improved skin health to increased muscle strength.

The Multilayered Marvel: Skin Anatomy

Human skin is a complex organ with three primary layers:

1. **Epidermis:** The skin's outermost layer is made up of

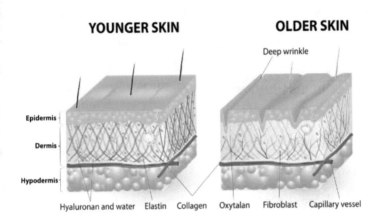

YOUNGER SKIN   **OLDER SKIN**

Deep wrinkle

Epidermis
Dermis
Hypodermis

Hyaluronan and water   Elastin   Collagen   Oxytalan   Fibroblast   Capillary vessel

sub-layers, namely the stratum corneum, stratum lucidum, stratum granulosum, stratum spinosum, and stratum basale. Collectively, they form a protective barrier against environmental hazards, regulate water loss, and determine skin color through melanocytes.

2. Dermis: Beneath the epidermis, this layer contains various structures like hair follicles, sweat glands, and fibroblasts. Importantly, the dermis houses collagen and elastin fibers, which grant the skin its elasticity and structural integrity. Sensory receptors here also allow us to sense touch, pain, and temperature.

3. Hypodermis: The skin's deepest layer contains fat and connective tissue. It serves to insulate, cushion joints and organs, and store energy. This layer is rich in nerves and blood vessels.

It's essential to note that the skin's layers and functions may vary across different regions of the body. For example, the skin beneath the eyes is markedly thinner than that on the cheeks.

The Collagen Family: Different Types and Their Roles

Collagen is not a monolithic entity. There are distinct types, each with specific roles:

- **Type 1 Collagen:** The most abundant, it strengthens bones, tendons, skin, and other connective tissues.

- **Type 2 Collagen:** Found primarily in cartilage, it provides elasticity and cushioning.

- **Type 3 Collagen:** Present in the skin, blood vessels, and connective tissues, this type often works alongside Type 1 collagen.

- **Type 4 Collagen:** Located in basement membranes, it acts as a barrier and filters substances between tissues.

- **Type 5 Collagen:** Found on cell surfaces and hair, it often coexists with Type 1 collagen in tissues like skin.

Collagen Absorption: Essential Nutrients

To effectively absorb and synthesize collagen, our bodies require a combination of amino acids such as proline, glycine, and hydroxyproline. When these amino acids come together, they form slender protein fibers. With the addition of essential nutrients like zinc, vitamin C, copper, and manganese, our body can craft the distinctive triple helix structure of collagen fibrils. When considering supplementation, adults might typically consume 8 milligrams (mg) of zinc daily (with men requiring up to 11 mg) and between 3-6 mg of boron.

In Conclusion

Chapter 1 demystifies collagen, illuminating its integral role in the human body. As a cornerstone of our connective tissues and organs, understanding collagen's nuances is pivotal for anyone delving into its health benefits or considering collagen-based products. This groundwork is essential as we delve deeper into the multifaceted world of collagen in the subsequent chapters.

CHAPTER 2

Sources of Collagen

Collagen plays an indispensable role in maintaining the elasticity and strength of our skin, as well as the health of our joints and other connective tissues. But where does this protein powerhouse originate? This chapter takes you on a journey through the diverse sources of collagen, its extraction, production, and processing.

Introduction to Collagen Absorption

Collagen in its intact form cannot be directly absorbed by our bodies. To enable its entry into the bloodstream, it must first be broken down into peptides. These peptides, in turn, are further broken down into the amino acids that constitute proteins like keratin, essential for the formation of skin, hair, and nails. Most supplements often contain hydrolyzed collagen, the purest and most broken-down form, to ensure easy absorption.

Animal-based Sources of Collagen

The primary and most renowned source of collagen comes from animals. Bovine (from cattle), porcine (from pigs), and marine (from fish) sources are prevalent. For extraction, various parts of these animals like bones, skin, and tendons, known to be collagen-rich, are used. Different extraction methods, such as acid extraction for skins and enzymatic methods for delicate tissues like tendons, are employed.

Plant-based Collagen Alternatives

With an increasing demand for vegetarian and vegan alternatives, plant-based sources of collagen, such as seaweed and specific mushroom varieties, have gained traction. While they serve the vegan and vegetarian demographic well, it's worth noting that they might not match the protein profile of animal-based collagen. The extraction from these plant sources involves techniques like water extraction and fermentation. Notably, fermentation has

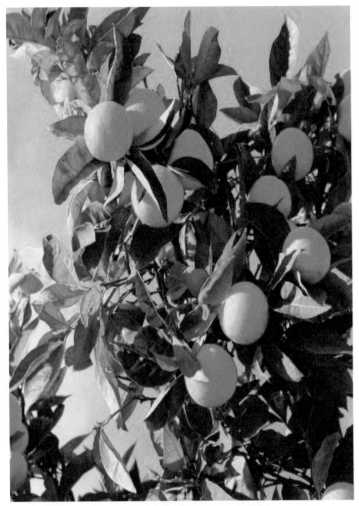

shown effectiveness in releasing valuable collagen components.

Interestingly, when discussing collagen production, it's essential to highlight the role of vitamin C. Oranges, a prominent source of vitamin C, play a pivotal role in collagen synthesis. Vitamin

C helps in hydroxylation, a critical step in collagen production, ensuring that skin remains vibrant, resilient, and youthful.

However, consumers should be aware of various chemicals applied to non-organic oranges. One such chemical, **Thiabendazole (TBZ)**, is used as a fungicide to control various molds. **Sodium Orthophenylphenate (SOPP)** also acts as a fungicide to deter rot and molds. Then there's **Sodium Hypochlorite**, an ingredient found in most liquid household bleaches, utilized for postharvest chlorination, algicide, disinfectant, and as a sanitizer. This chemical, though, is also approved for use in organic postharvest systems under the USDA National Organic Program (NOP) Rule.

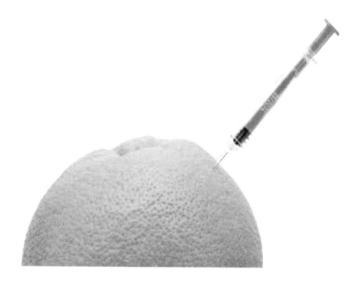

A compound known as **Maleic Hydrazide** is employed to induce dormancy in citrus fruits and control growth in various crops. An alarming chemical, **Sulfuryl Fluoride**, is a fumigant applied to stored crops after harvest, which leaves significant amounts of fluoride on treated foods. Several studies have pointed out the neurotoxic effects of fluoride, with associations found between fluoride exposure and reduced IQ in children. Additionally, sulfuryl fluoride is recognized as a potent greenhouse gas, drawing criticism from environmental organizations.

Another factor to consider is the artificial coloring of oranges. The Food and Drug Administration (FDA) has historically permitted the artificial coloring of mature oranges, especially in regions where climatic or cultural conditions cause the oranges to mature while still green. The coloring can be done by adding a dye, **Citrus Red No. 2**, or by subjecting the orange to ethylene gas, a process that hastens the blanching that typically takes place post-picking. Ethylene is also employed to "de-green" citrus, triggering the breakdown of chlorophyll and resulting in the orange or yellow hue of the peel. Consumers should note that artificially colored oranges might be adulterated if the coloring is used to conceal any inferiority or defects.

In summation, while plant-based collagen alternatives are paving their way in the aesthetic world, and vitamin C remains essential for collagen production, it's crucial to remain aware of the treatments and chemicals applied to food sources like oranges. Making informed choices ensures optimal health and well-being.

Synthetic and Recombinant Collagen

Beyond natural sources, the scientific community has introduced synthetic and recombinant collagen. These are birthed in laboratories using cutting-edge biotechnology. Although they can be custom-made and don't rely on animals or plants, their bioavailability and efficacy vis-à-vis natural sources remain topics of debate. Their production typically involves complex biotechnological methods, sometimes leveraging bacterial or yeast cultures.

Processing of Collagen

Once extracted, collagen undergoes rigorous processing to be made consumable or applicable. The transformation from protein to collagen involves multiple steps, ranging from the transcription of the DNA sequence for collagen into messenger RNA to the eventual assembly of mature collagen fibrils into larger collagen fibers. These provide the foundational support to various tissues and organs. The manner of processing can greatly influence the quality and effectiveness of the final product. Depending on its intended use, collagen is available in various forms such as powders, gels, and capsules.

The process by which protein becomes collagen involves several steps:

1. Transcription: The first step in collagen synthesis is the transcription of the DNA sequence for collagen into messenger RNA (mRNA). This process occurs in the nucleus of cells, and the resulting mRNA is transported out of the nucleus and into the cytoplasm.

2. Translation: Once the mRNA has been transcribed, it is translated into a protein chain. This process occurs on ribosomes in the cytoplasm of cells, and the resulting protein chain is known as a procollagen chain.

3. Hydroxylation: The procollagen chains are then modified through a process called hydroxylation. This involves the addition of hydroxyl groups to specific amino acids in the procollagen chains, which helps to stabilize the triple helix structure of collagen.

4. Glycosylation: The procollagen chains are also modified through a process called glycosylation, which involves the addition of sugar molecules to specific amino acids. This modification helps to ensure the stability and integrity of the collagen triple helix structure.

5. Secretion: Once the procollagen chains have been modified through hydroxylation and glycosylation, they are transported to the Golgi apparatus, where they are packaged into vesicles and secreted out of the cell.

6. Processing: Once outside the cell, the procollagen chains are processed by enzymes, which remove the propeptide regions from the ends of the chains. This results in the formation of mature collagen fibrils.

7. Assembly: The mature collagen fibrils then assemble into larger collagen fibers, which provide structural support to various tissues and organs in the human body.

Bone Broth: A Natural Source of Collagen

A notable mention in the realm of natural collagen sources is bone broth. By simmering animal bones for extended periods, collagen proteins are drawn into the broth. However, the body doesn't directly utilize this collagen; it is broken down into amino acids that aid tissue building.

Quality Assurance

When choosing collagen, it's crucial to opt for forms that undergo extensive third-party laboratory testing. The highest quality forms are free from antibiotics, pesticides, allergens, hormones, heavy metals, gluten, GMO, and rBGH (recombinant Bovine Growth Hormone).

A Deeper Dive: rBGH

rBGH stands for "Recombinant Bovine Growth Hormone", a synthetic hormone used to enhance milk production in cows. Its introduction to the dairy industry traces back to 1993, with the FDA's approval. However, several countries, including the European Union and Canada, have prohibited its use. It's essential to note that rBGH isn't the sole synthetic hormone in agriculture. Other hormones are used in dairy and beef production, and the declining use of rBGH doesn't imply the elimination of all synthetic hormones.

In Conclusion

Collagen, with its myriad health and beauty benefits, comes from various sources. Whether derived from animals, plants, or laboratories, understanding its origins, processing methods, and quality is vital for informed choices. Chapter 2 provides a comprehensive overview to equip you with the knowledge you need to navigate the world of collagen.

CHAPTER 3

Health Benefits of Collagen

Collagen, a vital protein in our bodies, offers a plethora of health benefits. As the most abundant protein, its significance spans from supporting skin health to maintaining joint integrity. This chapter delves into the diverse roles of collagen, its sources, the potential benefits of supplementation, and some factors that influence its levels in our bodies.

Do You Need Collagen Supplements?

While our bodies naturally produce collagen, this production can decrease over time. A balanced diet typically provides us with the collagen we need. However, the efficacy of collagen supplements remains a topic of debate, given that most studies on this

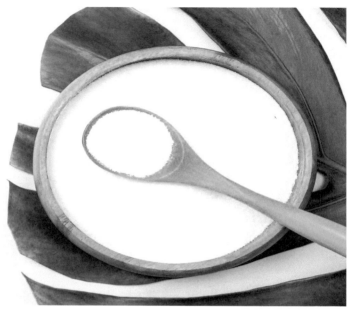

subject have been small-scale. That said, for those considering supplementation, it's reassuring to note that collagen supplements are generally safe with negligible side effects. They're usually available as powders, which can be mixed into various beverages or sauces.

Regulation of Collagen Supplements

Unlike many pharmaceuticals, the FDA doesn't regulate collagen supplements. This means manufacturers aren't obligated to prove their efficacy or safety. If you opt for these supplements, keep an eye out for keywords like collagen hydrolysate, hydrolyzed collagen, or collagen peptides in the ingredients list.

Factors Affecting Your Collagen Levels

Aging isn't the only factor that can deplete collagen. Sunlight, smoking, and sugar are significant culprits. Excessive sun exposure can damage collagen fibers, leading to premature skin aging. Similarly, chemicals in cigarette smoke harm collagen, resulting in sagging and wrinkling of the skin. Meanwhile, sugar intake can lead to tangled collagen fibers, making the skin less elastic.

Limitations of Collagen

While collagen holds numerous benefits, it's essential to recognize its limitations. There's no conclusive evidence that collagen can treat conditions like eczema, atopic dermatitis, or even acne. And while collagen injections may alleviate acne scars, taking supplements hasn't shown similar results.

The Veracity of Collagen Creams

Collagen creams, despite their popularity, might not be the most effective way to boost your body's collagen levels. These creams provide a barrier to prevent moisture loss but don't necessarily increase skin collagen levels. Comparing the absorption of collagen through the skin to pushing a basketball through a garden hose might not be too far-fetched.

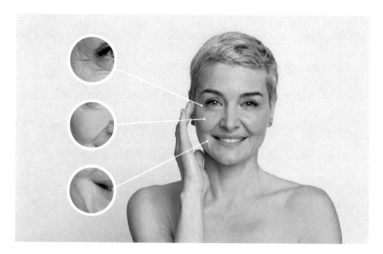

Collagen and Skin Health

Our collagen production starts to wane as early as age 25. This decline can manifest as joint pain, weakened muscles, or a change in skin texture. However, supplementing with collagen peptides can offer several benefits, from reducing wrinkles to enhancing joint mobility. Nonetheless, always consult with a medical professional before embarking on supplementation.

Benefits of Collagen Supplementation

For those who digest and absorb it efficiently, high-quality collagen supplementation can:

- Reduce appetite and support weight loss.

- Enhance skin health and reduce wrinkles.

- Strengthen joints and minimize inflammation.

- Counteract bone loss.

- Promote muscle growth.

- Balance blood sugar.

- Bolster hair and nail strength.

- Support vital organs like the heart, brain, and gut.

Collagen and Joint Health

Beyond skin health, collagen is crucial for our joints. It maintains the cartilage integrity, acting as a protective barrier. Animal-derived collagen, encompassing sources like beef, chicken, pig, and fish, can stimulate cartilage growth. This is especially

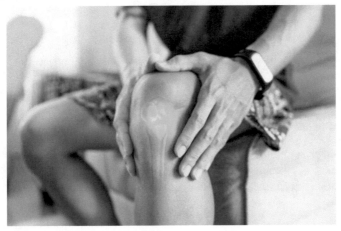

beneficial for those with joint issues due to aging, overuse, or conditions like arthritis.

Collagen, Gut Health, and Aquaculture

Fish are a rich source of collagen, but not necessarily from their flesh. Most collagen resides in other parts like scales, bones, and fins. However, it's vital to understand the challenges in aquaculture, such as the spread of sea lice and infectious microorganisms. Antibiotics are frequently used to prevent the spread of diseases among densely populated fish farms, which might lead to residue in the consumed product.

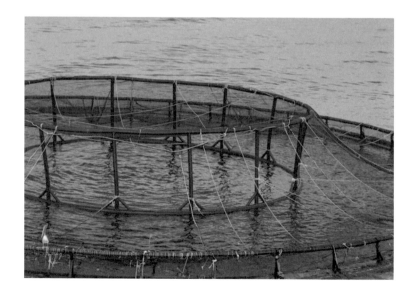

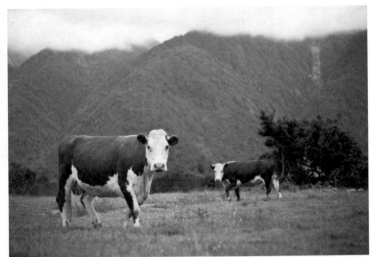

Sources of Vitamins, Minerals, and Other Additives in Food

While this chapter primarily focuses on collagen, it's essential to understand other elements and chemicals in our food. Several fungicides, growth inhibitors, and other chemicals can influence our food's quality and safety. Artificial coloring, for instance, is sometimes added to oranges. Moreover, Monosodium Glutamate (MSG), a popular flavor enhancer, has been the topic of various health discussions due to potential side effects. However, the FDA deems it "generally recognized as safe."

In conclusion, collagen holds a central role in maintaining various aspects of our health. While the body naturally produces it, external factors and aging can diminish our collagen levels.

James McHale, D.C.

Supplements and creams offer potential benefits, but it's crucial to approach them with an informed perspective, considering both their advantages and limitations.

CHAPTER 4

Collagen in Fitness and Nutrition

Collagen, a pivotal protein, plays an essential role in numerous facets of health, including fitness and nutrition. This chapter delves into the various benefits and mechanisms of collagen's influence on our body's metabolism, muscle building, and overall health.

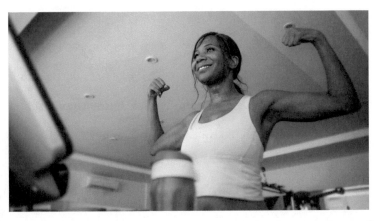

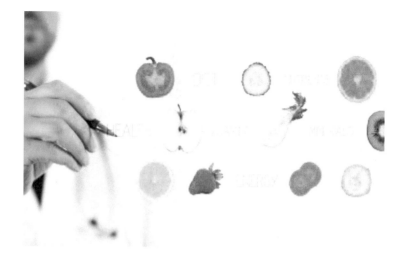

<u>Does Collagen Support Weight Loss?</u>

Collagen, when integrated into one's diet, may promote satiety, leading to reduced hunger sensations. This is instrumental for those seeking weight management solutions. A prominent element in collagen, the amino acid glycine, facilitates glucose's conversion into energy and contributes to lean muscle development. The rationale here is straightforward: more lean muscle equates to a heightened metabolism, primarily because muscles are more calorically expensive to maintain than fat. Furthermore, supplementing your diet with bioavailable zinc citrate, vitamin C, orotic acid, and boron can bolster this collagen-induced metabolic process. Particularly noteworthy is zinc orotate, an effective mineral transporter that facilitates the delivery of essential minerals directly into cells, optimizing their function.

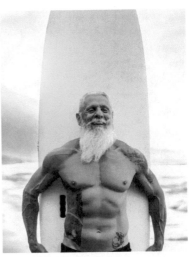

Muscle Building and Recovery

While both whey and collagen have demonstrated efficacy in supporting muscle growth post-strength training, whey might hold a slight edge due to its high leucine concentration. Nevertheless, to fully harness the benefits of whey, it's imperative to incorporate protease, an enzyme essential for breaking down proteins from cow's dairy, to ensure optimal digestion.

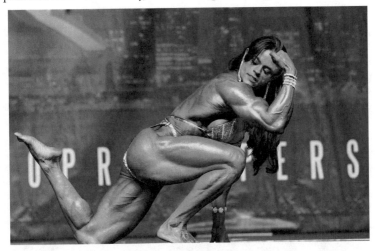

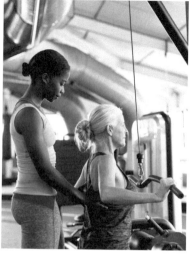

Conversely, collagen offers a unique benefit in maintaining a positive nitrogen balance, pivotal for muscle recovery and growth. An imbalance, particularly a negative one, often indicates malnourishment or excessive strain on the body, potentially leading to muscle wastage. Additionally, collagen strengthens the muscle cells' extra-cellular matrix, allowing for effective force distribution during strenuous activities without necessarily increasing muscle size. This property of collagen has attracted the attention of research-ers, with numerous studies corroborating its efficacy in improving

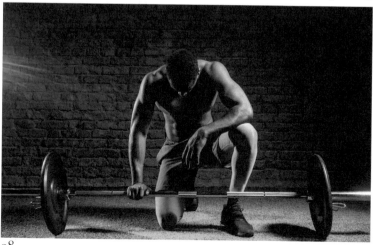

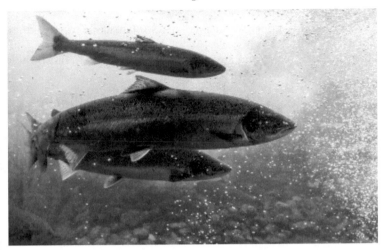

body composition and muscle strength across diverse populations, from seniors to elite athletes.

Foods to Boost Your Collagen Levels

Our dietary choices can naturally enhance our body's collagen production. The synthesis of collagen requires amino acids like glycine and proline, abundantly found in high-protein foods like chicken, fish, beef, eggs, dairy, and beans. Moreover, other essential nutrients like vitamin

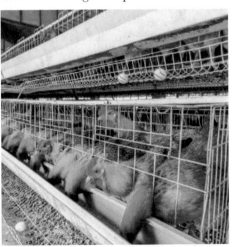

C, zinc, and copper play a pivotal role. Citrus fruits, tomatoes, and leafy greens are rich in vitamin C, while shellfish, nuts, whole grains, and beans provide ample zinc and copper.

Clinical Insights and Recommendations

Over a decade and a half of research indicates that integrating collagen peptides, a form of collagen processed through hydrolysis, into our daily diet can confer numerous health benefits. Notably, while collagen protein may be considered an "incomplete" source due to the absence of tryptophan, it still offers an array of active peptides and vital amino acids that can enhance health, especially concerning the demands of aging and rigorous physical activity. A study utilizing the PDCAAS methodology indicated that up to 36% of dietary collagen peptides could be incorporated into a standard American diet without compromising essential amino acid requirements. This suggests that the commonly recommended dosages of collagen peptides, ranging from 2.5 to 15 g daily, are well within safe and effective consumption limits.

Case Study

1. Introduction

Functional foods provide health benefits beyond basic nutrition [1]. The primary role of the diet is to provide sufficient nutrients to meet the nutritional requirements of an individual. However, nutrition science has advanced from the classical concepts of avoiding nutrient deficiencies and basic nutritional adequacy to the concept of optimal health, with the research focus shifting to the identification of biologically active components in foods with potential health benefits or desirable physiological effects [2].

Food-derived bioactive peptides are a product of the hydrolysis of the parent protein source, resulting in specific amino acid sequences that exert positive physiological effects on the body, often distinct from the effects of the individual amino acids they contain. Bioactive peptides are inactive within the native protein, but once cleaved from the native protein by digestion, fermentation, or specific processing, they are shown to produce beneficial effects relating to optimal physical and mental well-being and may also reduce the risk of disease [3,4].

Collagen is a well-established source of functional peptides with biological activity [5]. As functional foods, collagen peptides have been shown to exhibit important physiological functions with a positive impact on health. Numerous studies have shown an improvement in skin elasticity [6], the recovery of lost cartilage tissue [7], reduced activity-related joint pain [8,9], strengthened tendons and ligaments [10,11,12,13], increased lean body mass in elderly men and premenopausal women [14,15], and increased bone mineral density in postmenopausal women [16]. These studies have investigated supplementation with doses of 2.5 to 15 g of bioactive collagen peptides over periods of three to 18 months. The benefits are explained by the ability of bioactive collagen peptides to upregulate the synthesis of extracellular matrix proteins in various tissues via a stimulatory cell effect while providing the specific amino acid building blocks for body collagens [17].

Evidence suggests that the health benefits of collagen peptides support the principle that incorporating such functional components in the daily diet would enhance whole body collagen turnover and other aspects of health more effectively than the current average mix of proteins in common Western diets [18,19,20]. Despite the low indispensable to dispensable amino acid ratio in collagen protein, the Western pattern diet usually contains a significantly high amount of indispensable amino acids, due to high intakes of protein derived from animal food sources [21].

The current method for routinely assessing the adequacy of

indispensable amino acids for a given food or diet is PDCAAS (Protein Digestibility-corrected Amino Acid Score), which is due to be replaced by the new approach DIAAS (Digestible Indispensable Amino Acid Score) [22,23]. Despite its limitations [23], PDCAAS has been adopted internationally in food law and policy. In the US regulatory framework, PDCAAS is one of the criteria for identifying and communicating that a food is a "source" of protein for food labeling and marketing purposes [24].

PDCAAS-based protein quality scores are used to adjust dietary protein intakes to meet the daily requirements of indispensable amino acids. Ideally, the amino acid scores (AAS) of a protein or protein mixture should not exceed 1.0, i.e., fulfill 100% of the indispensable amino acid requirements while minimizing excess. This is due to the fact that the body's metabolic needs include both indispensable and dispensable amino acids [22]. As a consequence, if one or more of the indispensable amino acids are present in excess of requirements, the diet becomes limited in dispensable amino acids, thus unbalanced, even though the PDCAAS remains equal to 1.0 [22]. On the basis of these observations, incorporating functional collagen peptides in the diet without compromising on the indispensable amino acid adequacy can add the nutritional value of dispensable amino acids.

The objective of this study was to determine the maximum level at which collagen peptides may be incorporated into the typical protein mixture of the standard American diet without lowering the overall PDCAAS score below 1.0.

2. Materials and Methods

2.1. Composition and Digestibility of the Standard American Diet

The amino acid composition of the standard American diet was obtained from USDA's (United States Department of Agriculture) 10th nationwide survey, the 1994–1996, 1998 Continuing Survey of Food Intakes by Individuals (CSFII) [25], which was the most recent to report on the average individual amino acid intake.

The digestibility of the standard American diet was set at 96%, as described in the WHO (World Health Organization) Technical Report Series 935 [26] (p. 96).

2.2. Composition and Digestibility of Collagen Peptides

The amino acid composition of the collagen peptides was selected from publicly available data on six commonly consumed dietary sources of collagen peptides—four samples from porcine [27], one sample from bovine (GELITA AG, Eberbach,

Germany), and one sample from marine [28] origins. The four hydrolysates from porcine collagen were produced using different protease treatments. The sample adopted in this study was that of the collagen peptide that resulted in the lowest proportion of collagen that can be incorporated in the standard American diet while maintaining a high dietary protein quality (PDCAAS equals to 1.0), after iterative PDCAAS calculations were performed for all six samples (Table 1). The collagen peptide selected was sample D from Ao and Li (2012) [27], and its indispensable amino acid composition is presented in Table 2.

Table 1

Outcomes from the iterative PDCAAS calculations devised to identify the highest percentage of each type of collagen peptides that may be incorporated in the standard American diet, while maintaining dietary protein quality.

Commonly Consumed Dietary Sources of Collagen Peptides	PDCAAS Equals 1.0 ("High" Dietary Protein Quality)		PDCAAS Equals 0.75 ("Good" Dietary Protein Quality)	
	Collagen (%)	First Limiting Amino Acid	Collagen (%)	First Limiting Amino Acid
Porcine, sample A [27]	39%	Tryptophan	54%	Tryptophan
Porcine, sample B [27]	39%	Tryptophan	54%	Tryptophan
Porcine, sample C [27]	39%	Tryptophan	54%	Tryptophan
Porcine, sample D [27]	36%	Cysteine + methionine	54%	Tryptophan
Bovine (GELITA AG)	39%	Cysteine + methionine	54%	Tryptophan
Marine [28]	39%	Tryptophan	54%	Tryptophan

Table 2

The PDCAAS calculation of the daily protein mixture containing 36% collagen peptides and 64% mixed proteins from the standard American diet, based on USDA's CFSII data from 1994–1996, 1998.

Indispensable Amino Acids	Reference Amino Acid Requirement Pattern* (mg/g)	Standard American Diet Protein Mixture			Collagen Peptides (Porcine Origin, Sample D)			Daily Protein Mixture Containing 36% Collagen Peptides and 64% Standard American Diet Protein Mixture		
		g/100 g	g/100 g Corrected for 96% Digestibility	AAS	g/100 g	g/100 g Corrected for 98.4% Digestibility	AAS	g/100 g	mg/g	AAS
Cys+Met	25	3.68	3.53	1.41	0.72	0.71	0.28	2.5	25	1.00**
Histidine	18	2.91	2.79	1.55	0.85	0.83	0.46	2.08	20.78	1.15
Isoleucine	25	4.7	4.51	1.8	1.61	1.58	0.63	3.44	34.39	1.38
Leucine	55	8.07	7.75	1.41	2.51	2.46	0.45	5.82	58.18	1.06
Lysine	51	6.97	6.69	1.31	4.31	4.22	0.82	5.79	57.92	1.14
Threonine	27	4	3.84	1.42	1.96	1.92	0.71	3.14	31.37	1.16
Tryptophan	7	1.2	1.16	1.65	0	0	0	0.73	7.34	1.05
Tyr + Phe	47	8.19	7.86	1.67	2.97	2.91	0.62	6.05	60.55	1.29
Valine	32	5.28	5.07	1.58	3.22	3.16	0.99	4.37	43.7	1.37

Cys + Met = Cysteine and Methionine; Tyr + Phe = Tyrosine and Phenylalanine; AAS = amino acid score; * Reference amino acid requirement pattern (mg/g) from DRI (Dietary Reference Intakes) 2005, for children above one year of age and all other older age groups [30]. ** This AAS represents the calculated PDCAAS of the dietary protein mixture.

The true fecal nitrogen digestibility of collagen was assumed to be at least as high as that of gelatine (98.4%) [29].

2.3. Iterative PDCAAS Calculations

Iterative PDCAAS calculations were performed on each of the six collagen peptides according to the guidelines described in the WHO (World Health Organization) Technical Report Series 935 [26] (pp. 94–95). The PDCAAS is the lowest value among all indispensable amino acid scores, corrected by digestibility and truncated to 1.0. The indispensable amino acid scores are obtained by dividing the content of each indispensable amino acid per gram of protein by the corresponding value from the reference amino acid requirement pattern. The reference amino acid requirement pattern used in the calculations was that of children above one year of age and all other older age groups from the DRI (Dietary Reference Intakes) 2005 [30] (p. 689).

The iterative calculations consisted of substituting part of the typical protein mixture of the standard American diet with an arbitrary percentage of collagen peptides as a starting point, such as 10%, and calculating the corresponding PDCAAS, which was equal to 1.0. The collagen peptide percentage was increased by 1% increments as long as the resulting PDCAAS was maintained equal to 1.0. This algorithm identified the maximum amount of collagen peptides that could be incorporated in the diet while maintaining a "high" dietary protein quality [22] (p. 43). In a separate calculation, the percentage of collagen peptides was further increased until the corresponding PDCAAS dropped to 0.75, which identified the maximum amount of collagen peptides that could be incorporated in the diet while maintaining a "good" dietary protein quality [22] (p. 43).

2.4. Collagen Consumption in the Standard American Diet

The average daily collagen protein consumption in the standard American diet was estimated by an analysis of the NHANES (National Health and Nutrition Examination Survey) data from 2001–2002 and 2003–2004 [31,32].

The Recommended Dietary Allowances (RDA) of protein for men (56 g) and women (46 g) aged 19 to 50 years [30] (p. 645) were used to assess whether the effective daily amounts of functional collagen peptides (2.5 to 15 g) observed in the literature were below the maximum level of collagen that may be incorporated in the standard American diet.

3. Results

The PDCAAS calculations determined that a level as high as 36% of collagen peptides may be used as protein substitution while maintaining the indispensable amino acid balance and the high protein quality score of the standard American diet (PDCAAS equals to 1.0). The PDCAAS calculation of the daily protein mixture containing 36% collagen peptides and 64% mixed proteins from the standard American diet is shown in Table 2. The first limiting amino acids were the sum of the sulfur-containing amino acids methionine and cysteine. The PDCAAS calculations further revealed that the maximum proportion of collagen peptides that could be incorporated in the standard American diet is 54% while maintaining good dietary protein quality (PDCAAS equals to 0.75). In this case, the first limiting indispensable amino acid was tryptophan for all six collagen peptides (Table 1).

In this study, the individual amino acid scores of the standard American diet ranged from 1.31 to 1.67 (Table 2), indicating an indispensable amino acid surplus of 31% to 67% that allowed for the 36% substitution with collagen peptides, while maintaining the PDCAAS of the diet equal to 1.0.

Figure 1 illustrates the differences in balance between indispensable and dispensable amino acids, when the total protein in the standard American diet is replaced with 36% collagen peptides. This figure suggests that enriching the diet with effective amounts of collagen peptides could contribute to a better nutritional balance of the twenty dietary amino acids, while maintaining the high protein quality score of the diet.

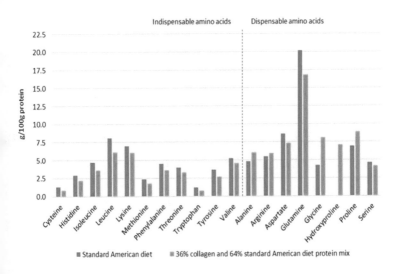

Figure 1

Illustration of the balance between indispensable and dispensable amino acids when the total protein in the standard American diet is replaced with 36% collagen peptides compared to the predominance of indispensable amino acids in the standard American diet. Absolute values are based on the amino acid composition of the standard American diet and collagen peptides of porcine origin sample D [27].

Table 3 shows the estimated average dietary collagen protein consumption, which varied from 3 g per day for those not consuming sausages or frankfurters in large quantities, to 23 g per day for those consuming these items in significant quantities. This indicates that collagen protein consumption varies widely according to food choices and dietary habits, which may significantly impact on the profile of amino acids obtained from the total protein intake.

Table 3

Estimated average daily collagen protein consumption in the standard American diet by males and females, using NHANES data from 2001–2004.

Main Food Groups Sources of Dietary Collagen Protein (NHANES 2001–2004)	Average Collagen Protein (% Dry Weight)	Average Daily Consumption			
		Males		Females	
		Food Group (g)	Collagen Protein (g)	Food Group (g)	Collagen Protein (g)
Beef, pork, veal, lamb, and game	5.15	70.87	3.6	39.69	2.04
Chicken, turkey, and other poultry	1.4	42.52	0.6	34.02	0.48
Seafood	5.5	19.84	1.1	14.17	0.78
Frankfurters, sausages and luncheon meats	55.43	31.18	17.3	17.01	9.43
Total, high consumers of frankfurters, sausages, and luncheon meats			22.6		12.7
Total, no consumers of frankfurters, sausages, and luncheon meats			5.3		3.3

When compared to both the minimum RDAs [30] and the actual dietary protein intakes for both men and women in absolute values [33], the effective daily amounts of functional collagen peptides (2.5 to 15 g) observed in the literature [6,7,8,9,10,11,12,13,14,15,16] were found to be below the maximum level of collagen that may be incorporated in the standard

American diet (Table 4).

Table 4

Effective daily amounts of functional collagen peptides (2.5 to 15 g) observed in the literature, expressed as (A) percent of the Recommended Dietary Allowances (RDA) for both men and women and (B) percent of the average daily protein intake in the standard American diet *.

		Effective Daily Amounts of Functional Collagen Peptides	
		Min 2.5 g	Max 15 g
(A)	RDA (g)	RDA (%)	RDA (%)
Men	56	4	27
Women	46	5	33
(B)	Protein intake * (g)	Protein intake (%)	Protein intake (%)
Men	100	2.5	15
Women	67	4	22

* Daily protein consumption in the standard American diet over the 10-year period from 1999–2008 [33].

4. Discussion

This study addressed the current challenge faced by food manufacturers and healthcare professionals in designing food products and communicating dietary practices for optimal health using functional collagen peptides in compliance with regulatory frameworks that are underpinned by the PDCAAS protein quality evaluation.

The study revealed that including collagen peptides at 36% of total daily protein intake maintains an optimal dietary balance of dispensable and indispensable amino acids (PDCAAS equal to 1.0). Any lower proportion of collagen peptides would maintain the high protein quality of the diet (PDCAAS equal to or higher than 1.0). When taking the amino acid variations in the peptide sequence of collagen peptides into consideration, which are caused by differences in food sources and processing, the estimated range of collagen substitution varied from 36% to 39%, based on the amino acid composition of the six samples of collagen peptides investigated in this study.

Relative to total daily protein intakes, the effective amounts of functional collagen peptides observed in the literature (2.5 g to 15 g) were found to be below the maximum level of collagen that may be incorporated as protein substitution in diets meeting the minimum RDAs for protein [6,7,8,9,10,11,12,13,14,15,16]. In practice, the daily protein consumption in the standard American diet is above the RDA, having increased slightly over the 10-year period from 1999–2008, from 15.6% to 15.9% (100 g) in men, and from 15.2% to 15.5% (67 g) in women, relative to the total energy intake [33]. Recent studies suggest that protein intakes higher than the RDA help promote healthy aging, weight management, and adaptation to exercise [34]. Should the recommended protein intakes increase, the effective amounts of collagen peptides will remain well below the 36% proportion of collagen determined in this study as protein substitution, ensuring that functional collagen peptide supplementation does not pose a problem of overconsumption. On the basis of these observations, effective amounts of functional collagen peptides would be better supplemented rather than substituted in the diet when consuming the RDA levels of protein. This approach would provide all the health benefits associated with collagen peptides while increasing total daily protein intake towards more beneficial levels and improving the dietary amino acid balance.

It is widely accepted that a balance between dispensable and indispensable amino acids is a more favorable metabolic situation than a predominance of indispensable amino acids since indispensable amino acids consumed above the requirements are either converted to dispensable amino acids or directly oxidized [21]. While human physiology includes metabolic pathways for dispensable amino acid synthesis from indispensable amino acids and other precursors, it is still unclear if the body's proficiency is sufficient to meet the dispensable amino acid needs for optimal health, which may become even more critical with aging, exercise, and disease [18]. Currently, protein quality scores are only determined by the indispensable amino acid content, although the 2013 report on dietary protein quality evaluation in human nutrition from the Food and Agriculture Organization (FAO) recommends that future research is conducted to determine the importance of dietary dispensable amino acid intake, and if there are circumstances in which account should be taken of the dispensable amino acids in calculating the DIAAS of a protein [22]. Also unknown is how the amino acid requirement pattern for optimal health differs from the current basic pattern, requiring more work to improve the general understanding of amino acid needs for different life stages, physiological conditions, and optimal health status [22,35]. New research in this area is needed to provide an up-to-date perspective on protein quality evaluation and categorization that considers the additional health benefits of bioactive peptides [22,36].

The lowest AAS of the standard American diet was estimated at 1.3, indicating a content of indispensable amino acids that is at least 30% above the requirements. Most Western diets have AASs equal to or higher than 1.0 because of high content of animal proteins that contain indispensable amino acids exceeding the requirements [21], and because dietary proteins limited in one amino acid can complement the protein sources that are limited in another amino acid.

The concern often raised with collagen protein is that a high level of collagen in the diet could lead to a low PDCAAS, mainly because of the complete absence of the indispensable amino acid tryptophan. In theory, PDCAAS equals zero when at least one indispensable amino acid is missing, as is the case with collagen protein. However, as collagen protein is never consumed as the sole or primary source of protein, its nutritional contribution must always be evaluated in the context of a mixed protein diet. As the adult diet is composed of a variety of protein sources, the use in isolation of the PDCAAS value of collagen is of no practical significance. This study showed that even though collagen peptides do not contain tryptophan and are low in cysteine and methionine, the average US diet contains a surplus of these amino acids that allows for the substitution of the total protein intake with 36% to 54% collagen peptides, while maintaining a "good" or "high" dietary protein quality (PDCAAS equals 0.75–1.0). An additional benefit of this substitution may be derived from the increased dietary content of glycine, proline and hydroxyproline, all major components of body collagens, which in turn represent 25–30% of total body proteins [37].

Analysis of NHANES data from 2001–2004 [31,32] revealed that the average collagen consumption varied from 3 g per day for those not consuming significant quantities of sausage and frank-furters, to 23 g per day for those consuming significant quantities of these items, a maximum of 41–50% of the RDA for men and women, respectively, and below the maximum 54% proportion of collagen that can be incorporated in the diet. According to NHANES data from 1999 to 2000 [38], consumption does not seem to have changed in American adults. Other dietary sources of collagen protein include aspic, desserts containing gelatine, or soups with broth from bones or cartilage. However, the collagen in these foods is not hydrolyzed, so they are unlikely to provide reliable concentrations of functional collagen peptides.

5. Conclusions

It is beneficial to include functional collagen peptides as part of the daily protein intake, not only for their bioactive properties but also for their rich availability of conditionally indispensable amino acids that may become indispensable under specific physiological situations and life stages. The recommended amount of collagen peptide intake may vary according to the specificity of the peptide (bioactive or non-bioactive), and to the desired health benefit (e.g., skin and nail health, joint health or muscle and bone health). The effective amounts of functional collagen peptides observed in the literature suggest intakes in the range of 2.5 to 15 g daily. These amounts are below the 36% proportion of collagen determined in this study as an adequate substitution in a high-quality protein diet, so that functional collagen peptides may be incorporated in the standard American diet while maintaining indispensable amino acid balance.

Author Contributions

C.P. conceptualized, performed the formal analysis and curation of the data, and wrote the original draft manuscript. S.L. and S.O. contributed to writing, reviewing, and editing the final manuscript. All authors read and approved the final manuscript.

Conclusion

In conclusion, the incorporation of collagen into our fitness and nutrition regimen can offer manifold benefits, from weight management to enhanced muscle growth and recovery. As with any supplement or dietary change, it's crucial to consider individual needs, consult with health professionals, and be informed of the latest scientific findings.

Study Source

Nutrients. 2019 May; 11(5): 1079. Published online 2019 May 15. doi: 10.3390/nu11051079 PMCID: PMC6566836 PMID: 31096622 Significant Amounts of Functional Collagen Peptides Can Be Incorporated in the Diet While Maintaining Indispensable Amino Acid Balance Cristiana Paul,1,* Suzane Leser,2 and Steffen Oesser3 Author information Article notes Copyright and License information PMC Disclaimer

Note: Some graphs/charts were recreated for this book.

CHAPTER 5
PDO Threads

In the dynamic realm of aesthetic medicine, new methodologies are ceaselessly brought to the fore, enhancing our ability to defy time and age. PDO threads, short for Polydioxanone, have emerged as one such trailblazer. Historically employed in suturing, these threads have now found a prime spot in skin rejuvenation techniques. This chapter unravels the intricate world of PDO threads, delineating their types, applications, and potential complications.

Introduction to PDO Threads

Aesthetic medicine has seen innovations galore, and PDO threads epitomize this progressive spirit. Not new to the medical

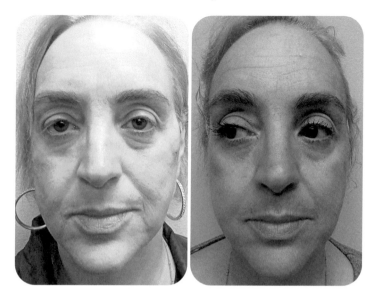

domain, their efficacy in suturing has been acknowledged for decades. However, their foray into aesthetic applications has been relatively recent. Their capability to rejuvenate, provide lift, and enhance skin texture has positioned them as a sought-after tool in aesthetic procedures.

<u>Types of PDO Threads</u>

The PDO thread spectrum is diverse, addressing various aesthetic concerns:

- **Monofilament PDO Threads:** Simple yet effective, these single-threaded tools primarily stimulate collagen production, fortifying sagging skin.

- **Barbed PDO Threads:** Characterized by tiny barbs, they deliver a robust lift to significantly sagging skin, simultaneously fostering collagen production.

- **Cog PDO Threads:** Sharing similarities with barbed threads, cogs have hooks offering additional skin support, making skin appear firmer and more youthful.

- **Tornado PDO Threads:** The next step in innovation, these twisted threads enable a holistic 3D lifting effect. Beyond the lift, they support facial and body contouring and promote collagen growth.

Uses of PDO Threads

Their versatility is one of the chief reasons behind the rising popularity of PDO threads:

- **Facelift:** Their most renowned application, PDO threads rejuvenate facial skin by combating sagging and reducing wrinkles.

- **Neck Lift:** Addressing the often-neglected neck area, these threads alleviate sagging, presenting a more youthful neckline.

- **Body Contouring:** Not just limited to the face, PDO

threads cater to body aesthetics by lifting sagging skin on the abdomen, arms, and thighs.

- **Scar Treatment:** By stimulating collagen production, these threads make scars, whether from acne or surgeries, far less pronounced.

- **Hair Restoration:** Tapping into newer applications, PDO threads are showing promise in revitalizing hair growth and scalp health.

Complications and Preventive Measures

However, like any medical procedure, PDO threads are not without their complications.

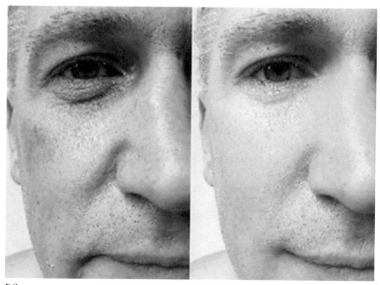

Thread Migration

Thread migration, leading to an irregular appearance, stands out as a potential issue. A significant preventive measure involves tying the PDO threads post-insertion. This technique, especially pivotal for barbed or cog threads, involves knotting the thread near its entry point, securing it further with sutures or anchoring points. This not only ensures the thread remains in its intended position but also promises optimal lifting. That said, the precision required mandates that only skilled practitioners undertake the tying process, minimizing risks.

Infection

Infection is a potential risk, as with all procedures that breach the skin. Manifestations of an infection include signs like redness, swelling, pain, and the presence of pus. The pivotal preventive measures include maintaining an absolutely sterile environment during the procedure and ensuring patients are well-informed with comprehensive aftercare guidelines. Should an infection be suspected post-procedure, it's imperative for the patient to seek medical consultation. A medical professional might then prescribe antibiotics or recommend other suitable treatments.

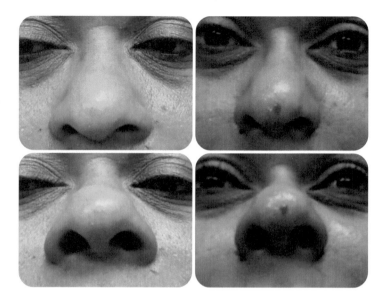

Swelling or Bruising

Another complication that patients might encounter is swelling or bruising. This is often seen at the insertion points or along the path where the thread has been placed. The risk of such complications can be significantly reduced by utilizing fine needles and applying gentle techniques during insertion. Some practitioners also advise using arnica gel or tablets prior to undergoing the procedure as a preventive measure. In managing such conditions, cold compresses have been found effective in diminishing swelling, while with bruising, a combination of time and gentle skincare usually helps in alleviation.

Visibility or Palpability of the Thread

A less common but concerning issue is the visibility or palpability of the thread. This is more frequent in individuals who have a thinner skin layer. Such complications arise primarily due to incorrect placement or depth during the thread's insertion. The selection of the appropriate thread type tailored to the patient's skin is also crucial in preventing this issue. If a patient does end up with a visible or palpable thread, professional intervention might be needed to either adjust or completely remove the thread.

Nerve Damage or Numbness

In rarer circumstances, there's a chance of nerve damage or numbness. This happens if, mistakenly, the thread is inserted too close to a nerve. Such an error can result in either temporary or permanent nerve damage, and the patient may experience sensations of numbness or tingling. To prevent such a grave complication, a deep-rooted understanding of facial anatomy paired with proper procedural training is indispensable. If a patient suspects nerve damage, immediate consultation with a specialist is essential. Based on the severity of the damage, various corrective measures might be proposed.

<u>Conclusion</u>

In conclusion, PDO threads have dramatically reshaped aesthetic medicine's landscape. From skin tightening to hair restoration, they offer multifaceted solutions with minimum invasiveness. As they continue to gain popularity, understanding their potential and ensuring their right application becomes paramount for both practitioners and recipients.

ABOUT THE AUTHOR

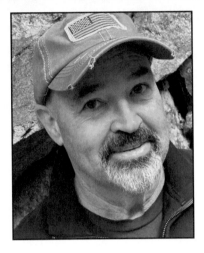

James McHale, D.C. has expertise in clinical nutrition, research, disorders of the musculoskeletal system, and aesthetics. With over 35 years of clinical experience caring for people as a chiropractor and previously as a respiratory therapist, he has authored numerous in-depth studies on metabolism, bone density, weight loss, and body composition. He has 2 patents pending before the United States Patent and Trademark Office for novel and unique surgical PDO threads for face lifting and nose modification. His interest in mineral transporter technology helped lead to the new collagen product he developed for maximum zinc, manganese, boron, and vitamin c absorption. That product is available for sale.

Jim lives in Bucks County, PA, and is passionate about nature, trout fishing, kindness, and second chances. He is available for seminars, workshops, and speaking engagements.

Made in the USA
Columbia, SC
03 September 2024

41138028R00041